Fungal infection

Laboratory Diagnosis of Fungal Infections

Dr Joseph Stanley

Table of Contents

CHAPTER1

Fungal infection

In most of the natural world, fungal infections are common.

When a fungus invades a human host, it can cause a fungal infection if the body's immune system is overwhelmed.

About half of all nail abnormalities are caused by nail fungus infections, making this the most common nail disease.

Although fungus is naturally found on the human body, it can become a nuisance if it multiplies too rapidly.

Onychomycosis and tinea unguium are two other names for them.

Infected fingernails or toenails will often change color, thicken, and crumble at the edges.

This problem typically manifests itself in the toenails.

Infected toenails affect about 10% of adults.

In this article, we'll go over the basics of nail fungal infections, including their causes, symptoms, and treatments.

There are both beneficial and harmful fungi, just as there are for many other types of microorganisms.

Invasive pathogenic fungi present a significant challenge to medical professionals due to their ability to persist in the environment and reinfect the patient despite their best efforts.

In this article, we'll discuss the risk factors for developing a fungal infection, as well as the signs and treatments available for several of the most common kinds.

Symptoms

Symptoms of a fungal infection are often noticeable changes in the skin's appearance and itching.

The following are some of the common symptoms of a fungal infection, though they vary depending on the type of infection:

• alterations to the skin, such as peeling or cracking

• itching

Keep reading to learn more about the signs and treatments available for various fungal infections.

Types

These conditions are all examples of fungal infections.

Ankle sprain

Athlete's foot, also called tinea pedis, is a fungal infection of the foot.

Because the fungus that causes athlete's foot thrives in warm, damp places like socks and shoes, sports equipment, and locker rooms, the two are often linked.

Athlete's foot is a common problem, and anyone can get it.

Warmer climates and summer months are optimal for its rapid proliferation.

Symptoms

An athlete's foot infection is common in warm, damp places where the fungus thrives.

Athlete's foot symptoms can appear red on lighter skin tones but dark brown on darker skin tones, depending on the person's natural pigmentation.

The classic signs are: • skin discoloration and blisters • soft, peeling, or flaking skin • scaling, peeling, or burning skin • itching, stinging, or burning sensations in the infected area

CHAPTER2

Treatment, prophylaxis, and diagnosis

Having athlete's foot is not the only cause of itchy feet.

To confirm a fungal infection, a doctor will typically scrape some of the scaling skin from the affected area and examine it under a microscope.

Athlete's foot can be caused by a few different kinds of fungi.

Depending on the type of fungus that has infected the skin, symptoms may vary.

In many cases, over-the-counter or internet purchases of topical antifungal ointments are sufficient to treat athlete's foot.

There may be a need for additional oral medications in cases of severe infections.

Feet must be treated with care, and kept dry, in order to prevent the fungus from spreading.

Keeping the feet clean and dry is an important part of preventing this condition.

Wearing sandals is recommended when using a public shower or locker room.

A fungal infection

Candida overgrowth manifests itself most frequently in women as vaginal yeast infections, which are typically caused by Candida albicans.

When Candida grows out of control, it throws off the delicate vaginal ecology.

Antibiotics, stress, hormonal imbalances, and unhealthy diets are just some of the factors that could contribute to a bacterial imbalance.

Diaper rash and fungal infections of the toenails are two additional common symptoms of a Candida infection.

Symptoms

Fungus in the toenails is often caused by a yeast infection.

Yeast infections manifest themselves through a variety of uncomfortable physical manifestations, including vaginal itching and swelling, vaginal redness and soreness, vaginal burning or pain during urination or sexual activity, and vaginal discharge that is either very watery or clumpy and gray, like cottage cheese.

Over time, a rash could appear.

Untreated yeast infections can worsen rapidly, so prompt treatment is essential.

Treatment, prophylaxis, and diagnosis

Yeast infections are simple to diagnose due to their classic symptoms.

When conducting a thorough examination, doctors may inquire about the patient's medical history (STIs).

They might also inquire about any recent antibiotic use.

Following this, the cervix and vaginal walls will be examined for signs of infection, and vaginal cells may be collected for testing if further analysis is required.

The severity of a yeast infection determines how it is treated.

Creams, tablets, and suppositories are the usual treatments, and they can be obtained by prescription, over-the-counter, or online.

Some infections are particularly difficult to treat because of their complexity.

Keeping a healthy diet and regular hygiene routines are the first lines of defense against yeast infections.

Loose, natural-fiber clothing may also aid in warding off disease.

Furthermore, changing feminine hygiene products frequently and washing underwear in very hot water can aid in preventing fungal growth.

Tinea cruris, or "jock itch," is a common form of fungal skin infection.

These fungi flourish in warm, humid places, such as the groin, buttocks, and inner thighs of humans.

It's possible that jock itch is more prevalent in the summer or in hot, humid climates.

The fungus that causes jock itch can be passed from person to person or from infected object to uninfected one through close contact.

CHAPTER 3

Symptoms

Men and women alike are susceptible to genital thrush.

In most cases, the itchy, red rash caused by jock itch will form a circle on the affected area of the body.

Skin in the groin, buttocks, or thighs may become red, flaky, scaly, or irritated; a rash with a circular shape and raised edges; chafing, irritation, itching, or burning; and cracking, flaking, or dry peeling of the skin in the infected area.

Treatment, prophylaxis, and diagnosis

Jock itch has a distinctive appearance that allows it to be easily recognized.

When in doubt, doctors may take a skin sample for further examination.

Jock itch is usually treated with antifungal ointments applied topically and a clean, dry environment.

Though some cases of jock itch require prescription drugs, many cases can be treated with over-the-counter drugs.

Fungus can also be eliminated by cleaning the affected area and maintaining a dry environment.

Loose-fitting natural fibers, such as the cotton underwear you can buy online, are effective at preventing jock itch.

It's also crucial to stay away from people who might be infected.

It may also help if you don't use the same towel or sports equipment as anyone else.

Fungus infections of the nails can be difficult and costly to treat.

Oral antifungal medications, topical ointments, and complementary and alternative medicine are all available treatment options.

There are ointments and creams you can buy without a prescription, but they haven't shown much promise.

Nail fungus can be treated orally with medications like terbinafine (Lamisil), itraconazole (Sporanox), and fluconazole (Diflucan)

Usually, these procedures take up to four months to completely remove the infected nail and replace it with a healthy one.

The entire nail may be removed by a doctor if the situation calls for it.

Natural treatments

While topical treatments for nail fungus may temporarily alleviate symptoms, they typically cannot eradicate the infection.

Also, other home remedies have shown clinical promise in treating nail fungus, such as:

Coughs can be soothed with Vicks VapoRub.

A study from 2011 suggests, however, that it may be useful in treating nail fungus.

Extraction of snakeroot:

Using this plant to treat nail fungus has been shown to be as effective as using the prescription drug ciclopirox, which is also antifungal, according to a study from 2008.

The thymol in oregano oil, which is said to have antifungal properties, is one example.

Oregano oil and tea tree oil are sometimes used together in treatments, but this is not without risk because both oils have strong side effects on their own.

• Ozonized oils, such as olive oil and sunflower oil, are infused with gases found in the ozone layer.

Multiple scientific studies have shown that this oil is effective in treating nail fungus.

Oxidized sunflower oil had better clinical effects than the standard antifungal medication ketoconazole, according to one study.

Natural remedies for nail fungus include Australian tea tree oil, vinegar, listerine, and grapefruit seed extract.

However, these products have not been backed by any credible scientific research.

CHAPTER 4

Prevention

Hygiene of the hands and feet is essential in the prevention of nail fungus infections.

Nails should be kept short, clean, and dry; socks should be changed frequently (ideally to fresh ones); antifungal sprays and powders should be used; hands should be protected from water by wearing rubber gloves; picking or biting nails should be avoided; shoes or sandals should be worn in public and around pools;

Picture Taking Precautions Include: Having Your Manicure or Pedicure Done at a Salon That Uses Properly Sterilized Tools Reducing How Often

You Use Artificial Nails And Nail
Polish Washing Your Hands After
Touching Infected Nails

PROFILE4 Roots

Nail fungus infections are caused by
microscopic organisms called fungi,
which can thrive in dark, damp
places.

Nail fungus is typically caused by
dermatophytes, a class of fungi that
includes Candida.

Trichophyton rubrum, the most
common dermatophyte that causes
nail fungal infections, is a yeast and
mold that can also cause these
infections.

The most common types of mold are:
• Neoscytalidium

• scopulariopsis\s• aspergillus

Nail fungus pathogens typically enter the skin through punctures or crevices in the nail or nail bed.

Fungi thrive in the warm, moist conditions provided by the nail.

Aspects That May Increase Danger

Fungal nail infections are more common in men than in women, and in the elderly than in young people, but anyone can get them.

Additional characteristics or risk factors for nail fungal infection include: poor circulation, slow nail growth, a family history of nail fungus, heavy perspiration, a humid or moist work environment, artificial nails, and socks and shoes that prevent ventilation.

Tight footwear that crowds the toes; exercise that causes repeated minor trauma to the hyponychium, where the finger tip attaches to the nail; walking barefoot in damp public places like swimming pools, gyms, and shower rooms; diabetes, AIDS, circulation problems, a weakened immune system;

Because slower nail growth and poorer blood flow go hand in hand with aging, senior citizens are

particularly vulnerable to nail fungus
infections.

CHAPTER 5

Ringworm

The skin infection known as tinea corporis, also called ringworm, is caused by a fungus that colonizes dead organic matter.

Both jock itch and athlete's foot are caused by the fungus ringworm.

The condition is simply known as ringworm when it occurs in any other location.

Symptoms

Jock itch and athlete's foot are both caused by ringworm, a skin infection.

The distinctive circular shape of ringworm is a reliable diagnostic indicator.

A scaly or itchy patch will typically develop into a raised, circular scar.

It's possible it'll spawn additional rings.

This ring's exterior can look red on fair skin and gray or brown on darker skin tones, and it can also be raised or bumpy, but its interior will look smooth and healthy, and its edges may spread.

Ringworm is extremely contagious and can be spread through direct skin-to-skin contact or by coming into contact with infected animals, most commonly dogs.

Towels, clothes, and brushes aren't the only things the fungus can live on.

People who play or work in infected dirt are at risk of contracting the ringworm fungus.

Treatment, prophylaxis, and diagnosis

Doctors sometimes need to take a skin sample to test for ringworm because it can look like other skin conditions.

Once a diagnosis has been made, the severity of the symptoms will determine which treatment option is recommended.

Many cases of ringworm respond well to over-the-counter or online purchases of medicated creams and ointments.

Some forms of ringworm, such as scalp ringworm or severe ringworm, require medical attention from a doctor.

Even the most fundamental hygiene practices can aid in the fight against and treatment of ringworm.

Maintaining a clean, dry skin care routine can aid in warding off skin infections.

Wearing sandals into public showers or locker rooms is one way to reduce the risk of contracting an infection from contaminated items or towels.

Aspects That May Increase Danger

Humans frequently contract fungal infections, but these conditions are usually not life-threatening if treated promptly and properly.

Fungal infections are more likely to occur in people taking antibiotics or those who already have a compromised immune system.

One's susceptibility to fungal infections may also be increased by cancer treatment or diabetes.

Prevention

Keeping skin clean and dry, as well as practicing general hygiene, can prevent most fungal infections.

You should not lend or borrow your towel, sports gear, or dirty clothes to anyone.

It has been suggested that wearing moisture-wicking, breathable clothing can help ward off fungal infections.

Repeatedly, people have been asking me:

CHAPTER6

Just what is the root cause of fungal infections?

The risk of developing a fungal infection increases when the body comes into contact with certain fungi and the immune system is already compromised.

An overabundance of the fungus that already resides on human skin is the root cause of many skin fungal infections.

Most people will get at least one fungal infection in their lifetime.

In what time frame can one expect to see improvement from a fungal infection?

After a few days of treatment, the symptoms of a fungal infection, like itching, may disappear.

Discoloration and scaling of the skin can take several weeks to clear up.

Can I expect the fungal infection to clear up by itself?

If left untreated, fungal infections almost never go away.

Actually, if you don't get them fixed, the problem could get even worse.

Outlook

The majority of fungal skin infections respond well to creams available both over the counter and by prescription.

More aggressive treatments may be necessary for particularly severe infections.

Fungal skin infections can be avoided to a large extent through preventative measures.

If you notice any signs of infection, it's best to see a doctor right away to prevent any serious complications.

Most cases of fungal skin infections can be treated with doctor supervision.

THE END

Made in the USA
Middletown, DE
05 March 2023

26235239R00022